LYDIA

LYDIA

*A Woman Who Defied
Operation of Her Gallbladder*

LYDIA

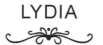

Printed in the United States of America.

ISBN: 978-1-4669-3870-0 (sc)
ISBN: 978-1-4669-3871-7 (e)

Trafford rev. 08/24/2012

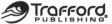 www.trafford.com

North America & international
toll-free: 1 888 232 4444 (USA & Canada)
phone: 250 383 6864 ♦ fax: 812 355 4082

CONTENTS

This book outlines my true experience when I became sick and got worst in August 2010. This is a true story and my journey of the following:

- How important to be Medicine-wise.
- How important to listen to your Body
- How important to be aware to different theories between the Naturopaths and Doctors.
- How I succumbed to the illness of 2.1 cm Gallstone

PREFACE

I WAS DIAGNOSED WITH A gallstone of 2.1 cm when I had my ultrasound at the Greenslopes Hospital in Queensland Australia after falling sick in 2006.

Later in July 2010 I got very sick again so that I could not eat at all for more than two weeks. All I could do was to drink water very slowly.

I was not sure how I got the gallstone but my diagnosis showed that I had in fact a very big gallstone. Perhaps bad diet or eating fatty food and moreover, stress triggers my gallstones because stresses can slow down the digestive system.

I was devastated by my situation. I thought it was the end of the world. But my faith in God and my strong beliefs led me to meet a Naturopath and, partnered with my common sense, alleluia . . . *I have recovered*.

It is my intention not to mention the names of doctors that I have consulted. In this book I do not intend to downgrade doctors; I have no intention in creating a revolution between doctors' theory and the naturopaths.

Nevertheless, all the people who read this book and find it interesting may perhaps be encouraged to be medicine-wise; to use their own common sense; to listen to their bodies and think carefully what is really good for that certain illness they are suffering from. After all it is our own body. I would be proud of myself if my book contributes good sense in managing our bodies for the sake of our well being.

MY WAY OF LIFE
AND LIFESTYLE

MY NAME IS LYDIA EXCELL. I am 56 years old and I was born in Ubay, Bohol, one of the many islands of the Philippines. I have lived in Brisbane Queensland Australia for almost 30 years. Even though we were not rich I had a happy-go-lucky childhood with my sisters and brothers.

When I was in my teens and twenties I was jolly, active and positive in every aspect of life. In fact I sang in every activity during my primary school and secondary school. My instrument and weapon in life has always been prayer and having faith in God in every way.

I remember my father had a small motor boat with a capacity of 8 to ten people. He used this boat sometimes for fishing and most of the time bought fish and crabs from other fishermen to sell as his livelihood, for his children to live on and to survive.

Like most of the locals in Bohol our family mostly ate crabs, prawns and fish with rice. Sometimes we ate rice with dried fish, 'ginamos' or anchovis and vegetables. I thought we were very poor because we ate crabs most of the time but when I went to Manila to follow up my papers to come over in Australia, I realized that only rich or average people can afford to buy crabs so my thought was wrong.

I studied at Ubay Central Community School in my Elementary School then in my Secondary School I studied in Holy Child Academy at the same Town of Ubay.

However during my fourth year high school I was asked by my sister Dina who got married to a man from Larena Siquijor to live with her. I agreed with my sister and I studied in my fourth year high school at St Vincent Academy in Larena and graduated there in my Secondary school.

Then after graduating my high school I went home to Bohol and during my tertiary I studied at the University of Bohol Tagbilaran City Bohol Philippines and took a course of Bachelor of Science in Secretarial Administration (BSSA).

Prior to studying in the University of Bohol Tagbilaran City, Philippines in the same year 1976 I also did a Medical Secretarial in St Paul's College in Dumaguete City, Philippines which was only for one semester with a duration of six months.

Looking back my whole experience as a young person I can see myself a very determine and gutsy person because everything I did was all in optimistic character.

Part of 1979 and 1980 I worked for the Governor's Office for a year then when a new Governor was appointed by the late President Marcos most of us were laid off including me.

After I was out of a job I was hired by a Lawyer in our town and worked for him for few months. I left working for this Lawyer when I got married in 1981.

When I was 26 I was still unmarried. Although there were five men who were interested to have relationship with me and in fact two of them were interested to marry me I seemed not decided to marrying any of them nor have relationship with them except for one man when I was seventeen years old but only just a friend. The reason for this, I think that it was not time for me to marry and I have not met my soul mate.

However I was writing to a young Australian as my pen-pal named Errol who to my amusement was looking for a wife and to make the story short after he courted me through his letter and immediately asked me to marry him it took me six months to accept his proposal of marriage.

Errol came over to Bohol to meet me on May 1981 and we got married on June 25 on the same year the date which was also my birthday. We were married in an elaborate ceremony.

When we got married, Errol was 28 years old and as I mentioned before I was 26 years old. Errol was a quite person and I was also lucky we got married. I considered it destiny to marry Errol an Australian.

You know why I called it my destiny? Because for me it felt right. We got along well. Although we are not rich Errol did not mind at all. In fact he was kind to my family.

So, when I decided to come over in Australia I said goodbye to my loving family. My father was so overcome. He did not know how to express his sadness. He simply shook my hand and wished me good luck.

That situation was difficult to describe as I was crying inside but I was only trying to be strong so I can hold my tears and my father will not be worried that I was really sad of leaving them.

I arrived in Australia and became an Australian citizen. I remember the first impression I have in Australia was a beautiful Country nice people clean and a multicultural Country. I saw different food which I have never seen in the Philippines such as Dim sims, Chiko Roll, Sausages. Honestly I never eat sausages in the Philippines because just looking at it

I can get sick I do not know why. The sausages I saw in the Philippines were small not like in Australia they are really big sausages.

To make the story short my diet changes from rice, fish, crabs, vegetables and dried fish to meat such as sausages, steak, prawns, bacon and of course with vegetables or salads and eating fast food and fatty food like red roster, cakes and ice cream.

At one stage my mother in-law served me breakfast a plate with 2 sausages bacon toast and egg. I said to my first husband where is the rice? I cannot eat this. So I just look at it. But I was told by my husband to eat it even though just little so my mother in-law will not be offended. So I just ate a little but after that I got sick I do not know why probably because my food intake has changed.

Then few months has passed by. I was lucky to get a job working in a take away food shop three months after arriving in the country. Then in 1988 Brisbane hosted Expo88 to commemorate the 200th anniversary of the arrival in Australia of the First Fleet. I worked in a food take-away there and had a wonderful time meeting and greeting thousands of people from all over Australia and around the world. Six months later after a final fireworks display the lights were turned out and Expo88 was over and I was out of a job.

Tragically in 1989 my husband died of a liver complaint. With this tragic happening of my husband Errol made me very sad. I could have gone back to join my family in the Philippines but I was determined to make a success of my life in Australia.

I decided to do some short courses to improve my job prospects. At first I did the 3 months course which was Receptionist at the Careers College in Brisbane. Then I also did a six months course called Managerial Assistant Course at Nunn and Trivetts College in Brisbane Queensland. This course I was told by the Principal at that College that it was in fact a refresher course based on my qualification I had in the Philippines. I successfully passed all of these courses and as a result in September 1989 I got a job working for the Queensland Ambulance Service as an Administrative Assistant.

Luckily, I was able to move on to working for the State Government, at the Department of Consumer Affairs in 1991 (now it is called the Office of Fair Trading which was and is still under the banner of the Department of Justice. My position was Administrative Officer.

Most of my daily life living in Australia was working. I rarely went out for the recreation or exercise that our body and mind requires to thrive.

While I was feeling the stressed at work I was also stressed because I was committed to sending money to my ten sisters and brothers to help them out and support them with their food, education and others.

In fact, I did not have much left over to spend on myself. I am still doing this even to this moment because I want them to be happy. Even though I am stressed out of helping them as it is not easy to earn money, my heart and soul felt so happy that I am able to help them.

When I was at work, I worked hard and focused to what I was doing. I did not even take morning and afternoon breaks. I think that was a mistake because it may have been a contributing factor in triggering gallstones. I have since learnt that our body and its digestive system require food and nutrients every 3 hours, even just a piece of apple and a glass of water is sufficient to have between meals.

It is important to make a regular habit of eating a piece of fruit or vegetable such as carrots or celery or apples and drinking plenty of water. *I now believe it will help me to become healthy in the long term.*

In the past, every morning I drank a cup of Milo and sometimes a glass of milk. I did not eat much. I ate one piece scone or muffin not realizing that this is not healthy to eat for breakfast. However I did eat lunch and dinner. For my lunch and dinner I sometimes I ate vegetables with fish or chicken and rice or lean meat with vegetables and sometimes I ate prawns with salad and rice. I ate red rooster during lunch this is twice a week. I seldom ate fruits I do not know why. I did not drink plenty of water I usually drank apple juice and sometimes drank a glass of coke or a glass of orange juice. Unlike my now second husband Nigel he eats a bowl of cereals with soy milk every morning and eats food for lunch and dinner like meat or fish or chicken with salad and vegetables but he never eat red rooster at lunch time like I did.

Also during weekends my husband and I always have bacon and eggs for breakfast. Mind you we all both have big serves of bacon and eggs with toast.

When we are young we do not think about what kind of food we eat as long as it fills our stomach and do not feel hungry and that's that. Now I realize it is important to have a strategy in eating proper food and drinking plenty of water or fruit juice **to avoid an early life illness.**

In May 1999 I met a good man and his name is Nigel of which I considered him as my soul mate and we got married in July 1999. We bought a house at Hemmant which is conveniently located next to the railway station only 30 minutes from Brisbane. We are happily married couple.

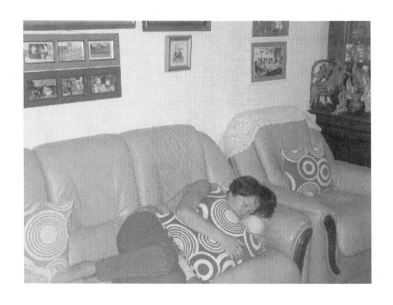

This is a picture during my illness

STARTING OF ILLNESS AND CONSULTING DIFFERENT DOCTORS AND NATURAL THERAPIES

I REMEMBER FROM 1991 THAT I usually go to the doctor only during the winter time. I consulted to my doctor about my flu and sometimes tiredness.

I did feel stressed sometimes however I felt really good most of the time.

Then after about 10 years I started to notice some pain and pinching between by chest ribs. It lasted a few seconds only but it was enough for me to feel dizzy. I had to stand up away from my desk and walk or do some light exercises for few minutes just very close to my desk. These episodes happened once or twice a week. I consulted with my doctor and I had an ultrasound and x-ray but no serious issue was detected in my body at that time.

I worked for the State Government for many years actually 21 years to be specific. I think because I was so diligent and conscientious in my work that I took everything seriously and I became stressed with the demands of my work. Perhaps, this was also another contributing factor to my gallstones. However I tried my best to adjust and not worry unduly about it. But we all know that everything has its limitation and perhaps we are all aware that stress can be a big contributing factor to many illnesses. I have learnt from my own experience it can slow down the function of the systems in our body. We are only human beings and no matter what we try to do for the best the results can sometimes turn out to be not what we would wish.

One evening in 2006 I suddenly felt dizzy and could not breathe. I felt a numbness of my upper chest left and right. I was really frightened of my situation. I do not know what to do as it was already almost six o'clock in evening. I prayed to God, please God help me, guide me what to do.

Then after my prayers I told my husband and I asked him to take me to hospital. My husband took me to the Greenslopes Hospital in Brisbane.

When we arrived at the hospital I told the Lady or the nurse that this is an emergency help me please. They were helpful although there were some Questions as I did not have a referral from the doctor. I continued explaining to them that it was an emergency matter because I could not catch my breath and was also feeling so weak.

I was given a small tablet by a nurse to put under my tongue. I forgot the name of the tablet. Then I had to take Panadol because the small tablet gave me headache. When I took the Panadol the headache was gone.

That evening the doctor examined me. I had the usual physical check-up including blood and urine tests. But I was kept in overnight and over the next two days I had an ECG, (Electrocardiogram) and X-rays on my chest and my upper back. I had ultrasound and then I exercised on a treadmill to try to determine what really triggered my dizziness and weakness as well as numbness of my upper chest.

The result indicated my heart was alright. However the doctor told me that it was appropriate for me to stay at the hospital for 2 or 3 days for observation. I was really bored as I stayed at the hospital just for observation. I was lonely and was worried what will happen to me.

There were many bad thoughts inside my mind. I was also missing my family in the Philippines. There were some questions in myself such as who will care for my husband?—My sisters and brothers as they all depend on me? You know—some crazy thoughts.

After 2 days of staying at the hospital the doctor came to visit me. He told me they could find nothing wrong with me apart from a large gallstone and the *only way to overcome this was an operation to remove my gallbladder. I was devastated and really worrie*d. I told the doctor that I did not feel any pain below my last right rib but only rarely the pinching that made me weak and dizzy and numbness in my upper chest. I told the doctor I did not want an operation; I certainly did not want my gallbladder be removed. **That was my decision. The doctor could not force me. However the doctor gave me his business card just in case I will change my mind.**

Unfortunately for him I did not change my mind.

On the two and a half day I was at the hospital I was told that I must have a stress test. I told the Doctor that I wanted to go home. He agreed, but he told me "before you go home you must have a stress test.

Ohh . . . that afternoon the nurse came and with a wheel chair and she told me to hop in. I told the nurse No, I am capable of walking downstairs. The nurse insisted. She told me that it is the hospital's policy not to allow the patient to walk downstairs. I was really sad and helpless that I have to be on a wheel chair. That was the first time and of course would be the last being on a wheel chair. I felt awful and lifeless.

As we arrived downstairs and after my stress test it happened that the nurse went somewhere. However she told me to wait for her.

Oh . . . No . . . no . . . no . . . I never waited for the nurse. As soon as the stress test was over I run upstairs and went to my room, packed my things and waited for my husband to pick me from his work. Then the nurse came to my room. She asked me why didn't you wait for me? I said I do not like to be treated like I am a disabled person not in a million years. The nurse was just looking at me and she walked away.

I was trying to defy my illness by my prayers. However I continued to experience the same dizziness and numbness and pains of my shoulder blades two to three times a week.

Because of this, I decided to see a Physiotherapist once a week for 6 months. I also started to have a massage once a week.

By 2010 I had to accept that I was just getting worse.

At work it affected my presence as I sometimes I have to be absent for work because I could not bear my illness. The way I got numbness of my upper chest and choking of my throat along with fatigue it wore me down. Sometimes I felt guilty to not going to work but what can I do?

I am a person that I do not like absences at all. I prefer to be at work rather than staying at home but with my situation I cannot help it and I was helpless.

Ultrasound result shows
I have 2.1 cm gallstone

Re:Mrs Lydia Excell
60/19 DOUGHBOY
PARADE
HEMMANT QLD 4174
PAT ID: 1155555

DOB: 25/06/1955
Our Ref: 1707770-1
Report Date: 12/11/2010
Service Date: 12 November 2010

ABDOMINAL ULTRASOUND

Clinical Details:
Large gallstones diagnosed in ultrasound performed in 2006. Ongoing dyspepsia ?GORD.

Findings:
Pancreas appears normal. Abdominal aorta is normal in calibre. No focal liver lesion seen. There is a 2.1cm calcific gallstone with wall-echo-shadow appearance. Patient is not tender to probe pressure in the region of the gallbladder. Common duct measures 5.4mm which is within normal range. The kidneys and spleen are normal.

Impression:
Cholelithiasis with wall-echo-shadow appearance.

Thank you for referring this patient.

CLOSE TO MAKING DECISION TO HAVE AN OPERATION OF MY GALLBLADDER

IN JULY 2010 I SUDDENLY got worse. I was feeling very sick and decided to have a break for few weeks from work. But then in the middle of August I could not eat for more than two weeks as it was too difficult for me to swallow. I experienced burping, choking, and numbness of my upper chest both left and right. I experienced having short breathes. I experienced sleepless nights. I experienced pain in my shoulder blades. It was a devastating situation for me. I felt that it was the end of the world. This feeling of hopelessness was so frightening—believed me or not it was so frightening.

I went to different doctors and they thought it was Gord (Gastro-Oesophageal Reflux Disease). Three of the doctors prescribed me tablets for reflux but I did not take any of them. I googled the names of the tablets on the internet. I was concerned about the side effects and also I was convinced that it was not Gord at all. I was right it was not Gord.

My illness and worry were exhausting me and I decided to take a total break from work. I felt I needed to have one year off. I was sure that after a year I could always go back to the work force.

I was obviously feeling really hungry but at times I could not swallow anything. I did not know what to do other than to keep on praying and asking for help from God.

Suddenly I had a mental image that I must eat apples. I tried to eat the apple and tried to swallow and to my surprise I was able to swallow the apples but only after chewing them very finely. Mind you it took me more than 2 hours to eat 1 apple.

Although I had difficulty in eating the apple but at least I had eaten something. Imagine from midst of September 2010 to November 2010 I live with apples and water. However it was better compared at the time from midst of August 2010 to the second week of September that I was not able to eat all. I live with my prayers and trusting God.

In few occasions I went to the city of Brisbane and looked at the people at the food court enjoying their food, I said to myself I wish I could eat them as well. Will I be able to eat food properly again? It was a bad thought and depressing situation for me.

I tried to see another doctor and in November 2010 I had another ultrasound and the result was the same. I had in fact a whopping 2.1 cm gallstone. In this journey of agony I also had numerous blood tests and it was frustrating.

Then I went to see another doctor in Brisbane City. I showed him the result of my ultrasound and he told me that I had no other option but to have my gallbladder removed.

I was really devastated and very confused. The doctor gave me a referral and the following day I had an appointment to see the surgeon specialist. I asked the doctor how he was going to operate me. The doctor told me it that it will be very easy to operate and remove a gallbladder and that a person can live without a gallbladder."

I responded to the doctor that, "even though I am not a doctor I really believe that the gallbladder is an important part of the digestive system and has important role in our body. *If my gallbladder is removed all the toxic can stay in the liver and in fact may go to pancreas and that will trigger another illness".* He told me that it *was not the case in fact he had his own gallbladder removed. I told the surgeon how about if you just take the gallstones instead of removing my gallbladder? The doctor replied it was not possible as my gallbladder is now rotten. The doctor also told me that if he will go ahead of the operation the result could be 50/50. (This words if I will omit mentioning in my book I could by lying to myself).*

My thought was umm . . . how does he know that my gallbladder was rotten when in fact he had not seen my gallbladder and in fact the ultrasound did not mention that my gallbladder was rotten? What a positive thought?

On the same day, the surgeon gave me another referral so that I could have another blood test. The doctor has told me that after this blood test he would examine me and prepare for my gallbladder operation as soon as possible.

To be honest, I did not even go to the Pathologist to have a blood test.

While I was still in doubt, the following day I spent the whole day doing research on the internet about gallbladder removal. *I concluded from my research that I was right and that some people who have their gallbladder removed still suffered the same symptoms.*

At first, when I went and saw the surgeon specialist I kind of agreed to have my gallbladder removed because I felt I have no way out.

But then I thank God he never forsake me and I found the way out. Yes, I changed my mind. I decided very strongly that I would never go back to see the surgeon and would not have an operation at all.

PRAYERS TO ALMIGHTY GOD AND RESEARCH

EACH DAY I HELD ON to prayers. I was crying when I prayed to God for help. I have a little altar in our house and I kneeled and pray so hard to God. When I pray I prayed in our language which is Visayan language. I focus mentioning my illness when I prayed. Prayer: "Oh Langitnon ug maloloy on nga Dios Amahan malooy ka kanako tangtangi ako sa akong sakit. Hinloi and akong gallbladder ug pagawasa ang mga gallstones nga walay complikasyon" Tagai ako ug kabaskog sa lawas ug hataas ug malipayon nga kinabuhi Dios ko, Amen. Prayer Interpretation in English: "Oh Heavenly Father, have mercy on me. Please root out the gallstones and cleanse my gallbladder without complication. Restore me to full good health and give me a long and happy life Oh Lord, Amen." This prayer I kept on repeating every minute and every hour whether I have to kneel in front of my small altar or pray in silence wherever I go or wherever I went.

I also continued doing research on the internet and found that, there are in fact many ways of breaking up the gallstone so that it may pass from the gallbladder. I never tried any of these as my gallstone was very big.

One day I had to go into Brisbane to find further help. My husband was already at work. He did not know that day after he left for work that I was really serious as I could not breathe and the numbness of my upper chest had appeared again.

I was waiting for the train at Hemmant. I was really in agony. One lady was sitting next to me. I confided to her about my situation and she was really helpful. She looked worried about what was going to happen to me. She asked me about my husband's mobile phone number so if anything happened to me she can ring him. I gave her my husband's mobile phone number and she also gave me her mobile phone number. We both got off at Central station in Brisbane and the lady told me to ring her if anything happened.

As I was walking through the Myer Shopping Centre in Brisbane, I saw a herbal shop called Healthy Life. I went in the shop and without hesitation I told my problem to Joy, one of the assistants. She was really concerned about me and she told me that in that shop they had a qualified Naturopath, his name is Ben Kashi. Joy told me that this Naturopath may be able to break the gallstone. I said really? What if the gallstone is already big? Joy answered you just try this qualified Naturopath and see how it goes. I said to Joy thank you for your help I will think carefully regarding your advice.

Then I went home and was really hesitant to have a consultation with a Naturopath as I have never seen a Naturopath ever. I was confused first. I was kind of ignorant about Naturopath's capabilities.

FINDING A NATUROPATH

ON THAT DAY AS I came home from Brisbane I had mixed feelings whether to go back and see the surgeon or to make an appointment with the Naturopath. I was really confused and I felt I could not go on anymore as the numbness of the whole of my upper chest got worse and worse.

I cried a lot and seriously prayed to God. Then suddenly I rang the Healthy Life shop and made an appointment to see Ben Kashi the Naturopath. My first appointment to see him was on the 19th of November 2010.

I was told that he only come in Brisbane every Friday so I had to wait for few days as it was still only Tuesday.

Then the day came to see the Naturopath. When I went in to his Office I was very nervous. In my mind I was so afraid of what he would say after explaining to him all my symptoms. He then looked at my both eyes through a special lens. He looked at my tongue also and then he told me "I wish you had seen me earlier as your gallstone is so big." My heart was pumping so fast thinking that he would refuse to treat me as my gallstone was already big. If he refuses to treat me it means I have no other option but to have my gallbladder be removed by a Doctor that was my very thought inside my mind.

Because I really wanted to be treated by this Naturopath I told him "I think God has guided me to see you and that I will try my best to follow whatever I have to do during the treatment". Honestly, I did not even realized the words that were came out from my mouth stricken him with pity to myself.

The Naturopath said to me "We can only try our best and we have to trust in God. Whatever my instructions, you must follow carefully and be positive that you will be cured. *No negativity in any way*".

After hearing these words I was really happy. I told the Naturopath I will follow his instructions fully. It was kind of a relief and was also kind of mixed emotions as I kept saying to him "I really need something to take now as I cannot swallow and the choking of my throat and numbness gets worse". The Naturopath told me not to worry as he would give me some herbal medication as soon as the consultation was over. Mind you it took one hour just for the consultation. This was fair enough because I had so many questions for him. He continued to view my eyes as he could determine the full illness of a person by looking at their eyes and tongue. Finally the Naturopath completed the examination of my eyes and my tongue.

The Naturopath's finding that apart from my big gallstone I have in fact problems of my cholesterol. I had high bad cholesterol and also my hormones were low. I was happy then that I decided to see Ben Kashi the Naturopath.

FOLLOWING INSTRUCTIONS OF A NATUROPATH AND MY COMMON SENSE

I WAS GIVEN A VERY strict set of instructions that I must follow.

These are the instructions of the Naturopath for three months duration:

ך Everyday for 3 months, during my breakfast, lunch and dinner I have to drink a herbal powder 2 teaspoons in a glass of water three times a day.

ך I was only allowed to eat steamed or boiled vegetables. Any vegetables were fine but had to be organic.

ך Then I had a tablet (Duo Celloids) intended to break and loosen the gallstones. I also took another Celloids tablets to balance my hormones which I took 3 times a day. When taking tablets of different kinds prescribed three times a day, to me it is important to have a one hour gap before you take the other tablet.

ך I had to drink a glass of apple juice particularly made from organic apples three times a day and after that I also had to drink another glass of vegetable juice containing carrots, ginger, celery beetroot and apples, again preferably organic this is also three times a day. However if no organic fruit or vegetables were available it was alright to use the non-organic provided I washed them very thoroughly to remove the chemicals. Plus I must eat an apple after each meal as apple and apple juice has a big contributing factor in breaking the gallstones. This is also three times a day.

ꓶ I had to drink 2 litres of water a day. With the water I had to dilute one teaspoon of apple cider vinegar which can also help improve my condition.

ꓶ I was supposed to exercise 30 minutes a day but sometimes I felt so tired that I could only exercise 15 minutes a day. My exercises consisted of running inside the house, stretching and a little bit of jumping and deep breathing using my diaphragm and released it through my mouth slowly.

ٱ I was also instructed to eat an apple after each meal for 3 months. But even now I still eat apples after each meal just to make sure that the big gallstone will not come back anymore.

Besides the Naturopath's course of instructions I also used my common sense so that I could recover from my illness sooner. I introduced my own regime and each month I partly fasted for three days. This entailed eating 2 apples as my breakfast and another 2 apples for lunch and another 2 apples for dinner but still drinking apple juice and taking the herbal powder and tablets. Then during the third day I drank a glass of water mixed with 1 tablespoon of apple cider vinegar and 1 tablespoon of pure organic olive oil which I drank in the afternoon. I drank 1 teaspoon of crust garlic in a glass of water once a week. Drinking a glass of water with garlic helps reduce high blood pressure and, in some peoples' opinions including myself, helps to prevent cancer. As I had to drink 2 litres of water a day I also included a glass of water with 1 teaspoon of apple cider vinegar and 1 tablespoon of Manuka honey with 1 tablespoon of cinnamon powder which I drank three times a day in the morning, noon and in the afternoon.

During the course or my treatment by a Naturopath and from my own accord I also had treatment from an Acupuncturist once a week for almost 4 months. *It may sound that I really have tried my best to be cured but it is true I was determined to keep my gallbladder.*

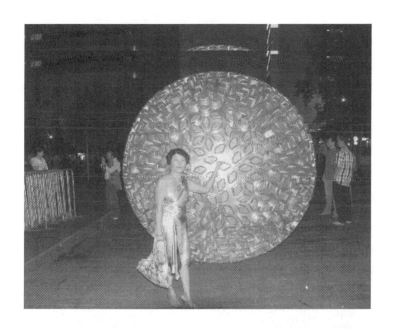

Photo after I recovered my illness

RECOVERING FROM MY ILLNESS

AFTER A MONTH I BEGAN to notice an improvement in my body. I could eat more and the numbness slowly went away and the choking and burping only came from time to time. Pain in my shoulder blades slowly went away. The tingling between my ribs began to fade away.

In this case, I continued taking the herbal tablets and drinking the juices. I continued to eat just vegetables and apples. To be specific I usually just ate steamed green beans and apples for three months. Mind you each time I went to the city because I like to eat hot beans I always go to that Chinese restaurant in the city at Cnr Adelaide and Queen Streets and requested them to just steam the green beans. I was happy they do not mind at all and because I told them also that I do not mind I would pay the same amount like I ordered stirred fry beef with vegetables.

When it was almost three months I was so eager to know if the gallstones in my gallbladder were broken into pieces and had passed from my gallbladder.

So, in January 2011 I decided to have another ultrasound. I went to a different doctor for this ultrasound. I did not mention that I had an ultrasound before because I needed to get an un-biased opinion. I did not mean that doctors are biased but in my mind it may create conflict between my previous ultrasound and the doctors may be wondering who is at fault in examining my gallbladder.

During the course of my second ultrasound I got the impression that the doctor had also noticing something that made her wonder. The doctor took a long time to check my body and actually repeated the examination. If I am not mistaken it took her 30 minutes or more to examine me. I was feeling a bit uncomfortable because of the duration of the examination. Eventually she told me that the result would be sent to my own doctor.

Then on the same day I made an appointment with my own doctor and the following week I went and saw him. He gave me the ultrasound result. I was really happy when I read the comments.

This is the comments and you can also see on the actual report that the *ultrasound result revealed there were in fact gallstones that had passed from my gallbladder without complication*.

I was right in my feelings because every time I went to the comfort room I checked my bowel movement and it was different colors. There were black, bluish, yellowish and a bit of dark brown. I also felt something moving downward inside my body during the passing of gallstones. What I had felt was heavy tingling from my last right rib then it seemed like moving downward, I felt nervous!

What was it? It kind like something pinched my right breast. Each time I experience tingling I have to run and quickly drank a glass of water with a teaspoon of apple cider vinegar with the mother. After drinking a glass of water I felt better.

During the course of treatment I have noticed that my bowel movement was constant. I have to go to the toilet at least three times a day. I was also feeling happy to go the toilet three times day, because for me, I felt it cleanses my inner part of my body just like detoxing the digestive system of my body.

From then on, I had no hesitation in taking the herbal tablets and followed the instructions of the Naturopath without fear.

To tell you the truth on the initial treatment I was frightened. Taking the herbal tablets left a big question in my mind, "what will happen if the gallstones get stuck and cause me discomfort, or worse still, create a serious situation inside me?" I was so afraid that I asked the Naturopath to monitor my progress. Luckily he agreed so I went to see the Naturopath every Friday of the week for three months.

After the result of my second ultrasound I went and saw the Naturopath. I told him that I had another ultrasound and showed to him the result. I thanked him so much. He was really happy also and he told me to thank God and he was also thankful to me because *if I had not followed his instructions the treatment would not have been successful.*

I also have to show the ultrasound result to my husband Nigel and he could not believe it. He said, "great, that your gallstone had passed without complication." My husband Nigel was so happy about the result. I told Nigel, "you know my dear, nothing is impossible with trusting ourselves and most importantly trusting to God the Almighty."

After three months the Naturopath changed my diet. I can eat fish. I preferred fresh salmon, I can eat bread but only multigrain brown bread, I can drink organic rice milk, I can eat any type of fruit and vegetables even when not steamed or boiled. I was not allowed to eat meat as fatty food as it were not good for my liver and digestive system because my gallbladder was full of gallstones and I am still on the way to full recovery. It is also understandable because meat is hard to digest. Although the main gallstones had passed I still have to be careful of what I have to eat.

I feel that after 11 months I have recovered from my illness.

I can eat anything. Even though my Naturopath told me to not eat fatty food even though I have recovered from my illness because sometimes I am craving for this I sometimes now eat cakes, eat meat twice a week but of course I still drink water mixed with a teaspoon of apple cider vinegar three times a day. I still eat apples and three times a day and drink apple juice one glass a day.

My illness and the problems and pain that I had to endure have taught me a lot about life and living.

In life, particularly when a person is sick, it is very important to be cautious, to do research. Now, that most everybody has computer, I urge you people to do research if you are taking medication please be aware of the side effects.

It is even more important to learn how the illness can be cured with natural healing. There is a temptation to take medication to be cured by a quick fix. But if the tablets have side effects that can trigger another illness *what is the point*?

It is important that if one is prescribed tablets that before they take them one should do research regarding the prescription. It is important that all of us should take control of our own body and our life in general for our own good.

In fact I know now that garlic, ginger, manuka honey and cinnamon are very helpful in contributing to a healthy life and of course eating plenty of vegetables, eating lentils, fruits, fish like fresh salmon and barramundi. Drinking plenty of water and fruit juices is also important for our bodies.

I decided to write a small book regarding my experience to let everyone know that it is important to be medicine wise and to listen to our own body and be in control.

It is important to seek different opinions from different doctors before committing to taking medication that is if you do not believe in **natural healing. You must remember that a quick fix may lead to another illness if you are not careful.**

Ultrasound result that I have succumbed from 2.1 cm gallstone

RE: MS LYDIA EXCELL
   D.O.B.: 25/06/1955

Date: 25/01/2011   3. Waiting

ULTRASOUND ABDOMEN

Clinical Details
Occasional brief epigastric pain.

Findings
Technically suboptimal study in view of patient's difficulty with breath holding.

There is an echogenic reflective interface within the gallbladder fossa. Appearances would be consistent with a contracted gallbladder filled with multiple gallstones although gallbladder wall calcification (porcelain gallbladder) may contribute to this echogenic reflective interface. There is no significant gallbladder wall thickening or pericholecystic oedema and the gallbladder was non tender with ultrasound probe pressure.

The CBD is mildly prominent measuring up to 8.5mm distally. No convincing common bile duct stones were seen. No intra-hepatic duct dilatation.

The liver, pancreas and both kidneys appeared sonographically normal. The spleen was partially obscured from overlying bowel gas. With this reservation, no obvious splenic abnormality detected.

The abdominal aorta is of normal calibre. Portal vein patent with normal antegrade flow. No ascites.

Comment
Echogenic reflective interface at the gallbladder fossa consistent with a contracted gallbladder filled with multiple gallstones +/- porcelain gallbladder. Mildly dilated distal CBD at 8.5mm although no obvious common bile stones were seen. Appearances therefore may reflect recent passage of a common bile duct stone. Are there elevated ELFTs? No signs of complicating acute cholecystitis. No other significant finding.

Thank you for referring Lydia Excell.

MY WHOLE JOURNEY OF THE ILLNESS TO RECOVERY

LOOKING BACK MY SITUATION IN July 2010 it was a very difficult and devastating time for me. Thinking now I questioned myself how I did it? Imagine every morning I forced myself to exercise. I prepared my food and prepared juice everyday.

I set up a time to take tablets. I also forced myself to look around at the Brisbane City three times a week because I felt it helps me a lot in forgetting my illness.

When I go to the City I always bring the food, tablets, herbal powder, apple cider vinegar and water with me. I always carry 2 bags. If I stayed home I lied down the couch not in our bed because I felt better lying not in bed as it helped me to think that I was not really sick though feeling miserable.

It was so boring and depressing situation but because I had set up a goal to break my big gallstone I have no choice just to go along with my goal.

Although I have spent so much money because of my illness I felt it was worth it as saving life is very important than anything else.

I hope that this book would give lessons to other people and I hope that you have enjoyed reading this experience of mine.

I would like to make it clear that different people may have different reactions but also, I am convinced that for every illness there is a cure and even avoiding an operation from that illness without the side effects is sometimes possible.

Although I have recovered from the worst of my bad health I am now careful of what I eat. I still drink juices but not three times a day but a glass of apple juice or a glass of mixed vegetable juice a day. I now eat more fish and vegetables instead of chicken or meat. However sometimes I eat chicken or lean meat but not more than twice a week.

Now I am happy that I was able to keep my gallbladder. I can now eat anything if I wanted to.

In my own opinion, without my gallbladder I feel that I would not have been a complete person. The evidence of ultrasounds that are posted in this book and my freedom of pain are enough evidence that I have succumbed to my big gallstone.

I have also avoided having an operation. I thank God, I thank the Naturopath, and to anyone who contributed to make me feel better during the course of my treatment.

Most of all I have to thank myself of my courage and determination in defying an operation of my gallbladder.

If I look back my situation during my agony it frightened me. Sometimes I questioned myself how did I do it? I know that the Naturopath tried to help me but I also knew that without my determination of keeping my *gallbladder I would have been a person now with no gallbladder and I am not sure if I can accept it longer knowing that I, in fact lost my gallbladder.*

I would like to warn everyone that they should not take herbal tablets prescribed by the Naturopath for my illness, unless you have consulted a professional or a Naturopath as each of us may have a different physical responses.

TIPS AND FEELINGS TO SHARE

BASED ON MY PERSONAL EXPERIENCE and during the time that I was ill particularly of my big gallstone I also noticed that I was in my menopause. At my age I felt there was and is still is changing life. When a woman or perhaps a man is in menopause era there is a feeling of different feelings in our body.

Personally I experienced sadness, also short breaths. My secret is I just exercised by running slowly inside the house. I eat plenty of lentils, green beans and especially if I cannot breathe I immediately drink warm water with crushed garlic and ginger. If I felt something was blocking my chest I immediately open my mouth and breath through it.

Apart from my big gallstone because as I had numerous blood tests one of the blood test results indicated that I had in fact lack of vitamin D and also lack of calcium. I was prescribed with vitamins that it seems would boost my vitamin D and Calcium but my decision is not to take these tablets because I was afraid of the side effects.

Therefore what I had done was every morning I did exercise. At 7 o'clock in the morning I have to open our garage. Our garage is facing the east and the sun just shines brightly every morning so when I did exercise I am facing the sun for 20 to 25 minute. I did this for three weeks.

With my lack of calcium I ate plenty of sardines and sometimes drank soy milk. The next blood test result was positive as my lack of vitamin D and calcium had improved. I also felt it within my body because from then on, I do not feel fatigue. I feel energetic.

So, based with my experiences that at the time we get sick that we should do something about it positively. That we should not just lie down we have to fight for it. We have to find a way to cure the illness before it is too late.

You know at the time I got sick there were so many frightful thoughts in mind such as what will I do now? Who will help my sisters and brothers? Who will take care of my husband?

This may sounds ridiculous because I was the one who was really sick and therefore they are supposedly to worry about me. However I cannot help this is the kind of person I am and the way I think life. I am a loving and family oriented woman. I care my family and my husband.

It also occurred in my mind that maybe if I was careful of what I ate and knew how to succumb stresses and/or maybe if I was aware what to do to be healthy then I would have done all those things. To be seriously sick is very devastating and sometimes I felt helpless to imagine my experience and what I had suffered.

Although I recovered from my illness it is important for me to be careful of what I eat and what I drink because there is a tendency that my gallbladder will be filled with gallstones if I am not careful. This is very practical would you agree with me?

With my experienced, I now felt how those people who had and still have illness like cancer and even mental illness suffered the pain within their bodies, soul and the spirit.

Sometimes I prayed and still pray to God to please help everyone and cure those who suffered illnesses as it is not easy to be sick. I pray to God to guide them what to do using their common sense lighten them up of the best medicine without side effects.

To pray to God within five to ten minutes a day can also help a lot but I guess I cannot save others as I am not God but I can only try.

I would also like to share this important story as this is about being healthy.

I have a brother who was *diagnosed to having diabetes.* He said it was type 2 diabetes but I am not sure because his two legs were swollen and the doctor advised him to stay in the hospital but my brother did not agree. Because I did some research about Diabetes I rang my brother that he should avoid insulin injection and other medication because the side effects are so dangerous. I told him that I will send him Bitter Melon herbal tablets and he has to take it as prescribed. I told my brother to eat vegetables, fish. He has to eat boiled eggs twice a week. He has to avoid taking sweet or sugar. He has to exercise 30 minutes a day just brisk walking. Above all I told my brother to eat fresh bitter melon 2 pieces every meal for six months. He has to eat raw cabbage every meal also. Most of all he has to drink two litres of water a day. I also sent him a cinnamon stick to soak it in a warm glass of water and drink it just a glass a day. The result was amazing. His two legs returned to normal. No more swelling. He now feeling good and when he had his last blood test the sugar level was so low. Well this brother of mind seems sometimes weak in managing his lifestyle because he cannot avoid to not to drink beer, or eat fatty food as he can easily be tempted by his friends.

Well, I told him he has to take responsibility of his own body and health in general otherwise his Diabetes will not go away. I cannot monitor him as I am far away from him. I am in Australia and he is in the Philippines. That's all I can advise to my brother.

To everyone, I hope that this tips and feelings I am sharing with you all will be useful and enlighten your life as life is wonderful. Life seems too short and therefore we have to make the most of it.

My theories are based on my actual experience not by experiments.

God Bless You All.

Important request: If you have read my book please send me an email on nigelxl@ozemail.com.au or write to: Lydia Excell Unit 60/19 Doughboy Parade Hemmant Qld 4174 Australia.

ACKNOWLEDGMENT

I am grateful to all the people like my husband Nigel who had helped me and Ben Kashi who treated me during my illness. They have contributed a big deal into my life.

I thank God and my courage to be a strong person.

Thank you for reading this book.

Author: Lydia Laboca Excell